DEFEATING ARTHRITIS WITH EXPERT GUIDANCE

Ultimate Solution Handbook For Patients, Guardians Or Family To Understand, Manage, Treat, Prevent, Reverse Symptoms And Live Well

DR. POTTER WHITLEY

DISCLAIMER:

This book's contents are meant to be used solely for informative purposes. The information should not be used as a replacement for expert medical advice, diagnosis, or care.

The information contained in this book is accurate and reliable, having been verified by the author to the best of his ability. Nevertheless, the author disclaims all express and implied representations and warranties regarding the availability, correctness, appropriateness, completeness, and reliability of the material provided here. You bear full responsibility for any reliance you may have on such material.

For informational purposes, this book may make reference to or mention of certain people, things, websites, organizations, or other names. The author has no connection to, endorsement from, or recommendation for these organizations. The author's approval or validation is not implied by the inclusion of these references.

Any direct, indirect, incidental, special, or consequential damages resulting from using or not being able to use the material in this book are not covered by the author's liability policy. For medical advice and counsel particular to their circumstances, readers are advised to check with experienced healthcare specialists.

The content, materials, and information in this book are subject to change at any time without prior notice, at the author's discretion. The text may contain errors or omissions for which the author is not responsible.

By reading this book, you understand and accept the conditions of this disclaimer.

THE REASON BEHIND THIS BOOK

In the field of managing arthritis, "Defeating ARTHRITIS With Expert Guidance" is a shining source of empowerment and information. This book explores the complex world of arthritis in great detail, shedding light on the subtle differences between its many manifestations and the significant effects it has on day-to-day functioning. This book offers a comprehensive view of arthritis, emphasizing professional advice as the cornerstone for successful treatment. It does this by explaining the subtleties of symptoms as well as the hereditary and environmental variables that contribute to the start of the condition.

This book's comprehensive analysis of the various forms of arthritis—from the more common osteoarthritis to the intricate dynamics of rheumatoid arthritis and ankylosing spondylitis—is a key component. It demystifies the diagnostic procedure while highlighting how crucial early diagnosis is to enable prompt action and better results.

This book's examination of treatment alternatives, which includes a thoughtful discussion of drugs, physical therapy, surgery, and complementary therapies, is one of its strongest points. The focus on lifestyle changes—exercise, diet, stress reduction, and sleep—highlights a comprehensive strategy for managing arthritis and gives readers the confidence to take responsibility for their health.

The insights this book offers on establishing a cooperative relationship with medical experts, encouraging efficient communication with physicians and specialists, and realizing the critical roles played by physical and occupational therapists all serve to further emphasize the book's importance. The emotional toll of arthritis is compassionately examined, providing coping strategies for both patients and caregivers and emphasizing the value of support networks and other resources. It doesn't end with medical interventions.

In addition, this book explores the frontiers of research and innovation, illuminating contemporary patterns and novel therapies that portend a bright future for those who suffer from arthritis. It doesn't hold back when discussing preventive measures, supporting healthy lifestyle choices, routine physicals, and long-term maintenance plans to bolster against the onset or aggravation of arthritis.

The inclusion of true success stories acts as an inspiring touchstone, which is possibly the most powerful aspect of all. Readers are provided with insights into the fortitude of those who have overcome arthritis by reading these personal accounts, which are laced with the wise counsel of professionals. By improving the quality of human experience, "Defeating ARTHRITIS With Expert Guidance" goes beyond the typical limitations of a medical manual and becomes a valuable tool for anybody wishing to overcome arthritis.

TABLE OF CONTENT

CHAPTER ONE

OVERVIEW
Knowing About Arthritis

A common and sometimes misdiagnosed medical ailment, arthritis is a broad category of joint disorders that cause pain and inflammation. It affects millions of people globally, irrespective of age, gender, or socioeconomic status. Arthritis is usually thought to affect the elderly, although it can affect anyone at any age and presents many difficulties for individuals who suffer from it. The word "arthritis" itself refers to inflammation of the joints, and different types of the condition, like rheumatoid arthritis, osteoarthritis, and juvenile arthritis, have different difficulties.

The most prevalent kind, osteoarthritis, is caused by the gradual deterioration of joint cartilage and frequently causes pain and stiffness in the joints. In contrast, rheumatoid arthritis results from the immune system inadvertently targeting the joints, leading to inflammation and possible abnormalities. The specifics of every kind necessitate specialized methods for efficient handling. In addition to its physical effects, arthritis can have a substantial negative mental impact in addition to reducing movement and making it more difficult to carry out daily chores. A thorough comprehension of arthritis, including its causes, symptoms, and variations, is essential for making well-informed decisions on its treatment.

Arthritis's Effect on Everyday Life

Arthritis has far-reaching effects that go beyond just pain in the joints; they affects almost every facet of daily life. Arthritis can cause stiffness and soreness that can limit movement, making simple tasks like walking, climbing stairs, or even gripping objects difficult. Due to the pain and discomfort brought on by joint inflammation, sleep problems are frequently associated with arthritis, which can have a domino impact on general well-being.

Arthritis also hurts productivity and employment because people must strike a careful balance between taking care of their symptoms and completing their work obligations. The chronic nature of arthritis exacerbates feelings of irritation, anxiety, and even depression, resulting in a significant psychological toll. Because of the condition's restrictions on social interactions and shared experiences, relationships may become strained. Because arthritis has such a profound effect on the quality of life, it must be managed in a multifaceted manner that takes into account the social and emotional aspects of an individual's well-being in addition to the physical symptoms.

The Value of Professional Advice in the Management of Arthritis

Managing arthritis is a difficult field that calls for more than a general strategy. It is impossible to exaggerate the value of professional advice when managing arthritis. Rheumatology specialists are highly knowledgeable and experienced, which allows them to create individualized treatment regimens that take into account the patient's general health as well as the type and severity of their arthritis.

Accurate diagnosis depends on professional supervision, which guarantees that the underlying cause of joint issues is found and properly treated. Rheumatologists are essential in developing treatment plans that go beyond simple diagnosis and may include physical therapy, medication, and lifestyle changes. Their knowledge includes keeping an eye on how the condition is developing, modifying treatment programs as necessary, and offering insightful information and encouragement to those who are afflicted with arthritis.

Effective therapy for arthritis necessitates cooperation between medical providers and patients. In addition to providing people with the knowledge to make educated decisions about their care, expert advice fosters a sense of confidence and control over one's health. In addition, continuous assistance from medical professionals facilitates people in overcoming the obstacles presented by arthritis, promoting a comprehensive and long-lasting strategy for arthritis management.

In summary, overcoming arthritis requires a thorough understanding of the illness, acceptance of how it affects day-to-day functioning, and an appreciation of the critical role that professional advice plays in developing individualized and successful management plans.

CHAPTER TWO

TYPES OF ARTHRITIS
Understanding Osteoarthritis: A Degenerative Joint Illness

Osteoarthritis (OA) is the most common type of arthritis, impacting millions of people globally. Weight-bearing joints, including the spine, hips, and knees, are the main targets of this chronic illness, which is characterized by the deterioration of joint cartilage and underlying bone. Even though it's frequently linked to aging, genetic predispositions, obesity, and joint injuries can also cause OA.

The loss of cartilage, the smooth tissue that cushions the ends of bones in a joint, is a defining feature of osteoarthritis. Bones rub against one another when cartilage degrades, resulting in pain, edema, and decreased joint flexibility. Usually, symptoms start slowly and get worse with time. While there isn't a cure for osteoarthritis (OA), there are several treatment options that try to control pain and improve joint function, such as medication, physical therapy, and lifestyle modifications.

For osteoarthritis to be effectively managed, early diagnosis is essential. Knowing risk factors, such as age, obesity, and joint problems, enables people to take preventative action. Moreover, osteoarthritis can be lessened in its effects on day-to-day functioning by exercising frequently, keeping a healthy weight, and shielding joints from undue strain.

Deciphering the Autoimmune Intricacy of Rheumatoid Arthritis

The synovium, the membrane lining surrounding joints, is the primary target of rheumatoid arthritis (RA), a systemic inflammatory disease. RA is not caused by aging; instead, it arises from the immune system inadvertently targeting the body's tissues, in contrast to osteoarthritis. This results in pain, edema, and eventually joint deformity in the impacted joints due to inflammation.

Rheumatoid arthritis is a chronic condition, which emphasizes the value of early diagnosis and treatment. For people with RA, prompt use of disease-modifying antirheumatic medications (DMARDs) can reduce inflammation, avoid joint deterioration, and enhance overall quality of life. Individual differences in treatment efficacy highlight the necessity of tailored strategies overseen by rheumatology specialists.

Rheumatoid arthritis can affect the body's organs and systems in addition to its joints. People with RA frequently experience issues related to their eyes, hearts, and lungs. Therefore, controlling the many rheumatoid arthritis presentations requires multidisciplinary collaboration as comprehensive care addresses the disease's systemic elements.

Psoriatic Arthritis: Handling the Skin-Joint Interface

Psoriatic arthritis (PsA) is a distinct problem since it arises from the combination of psoriasis, a skin disease marked by red, scaly areas, and autoimmune joint inflammation. People who have psoriasis are susceptible to this chronic inflammatory arthritis, which can harm the spine, connective tissues, and joints.

It is essential to comprehend the connection between psoriasis and psoriatic arthritis to make an accurate diagnosis and provide appropriate treatment. Because the symptoms related to the skin and joints might arise simultaneously or separately, medical professionals must perform comprehensive evaluations. Since psoriatic arthritis frequently mimics other types of arthritis in terms of joint pain, stiffness, and swelling, it is important to have experience differentiating between the two.

Medications such as biologics, disease-modifying antirheumatic drugs (DMARDs), and nonsteroidal anti-inflammatory medicines (NSAIDs) are commonly used in combination to treat psoriatic arthritis. Furthermore, lifestyle adjustments like stress management and keeping a healthy weight can help produce better results. A comprehensive strategy that treats the skin and joint symptoms of psoriatic arthritis requires cooperation between dermatologists and rheumatologists.

Revealing the Effects of Ankylosing Spondylitis on the Spine

One kind of inflammatory arthritis that mostly affects the spine is called ankylosing spondylitis, or AS. This long-term ailment results in inflammation of the spinal joints, which in turn produces pain, stiffness, and ultimately vertebral fusion. Although the precise etiology of ankylosing spondylitis remains incompletely comprehended, genetic variables, including the existence of the HLA-B27 gene, significantly influence susceptibility.

Inflammatory back pain is the main symptom of ankylosing spondylitis; it usually gets worse at rest and gets better when you move. Initiating suitable treatment measures to manage symptoms and prevent long-term consequences, like spinal fusion, requires an early diagnosis.

A mix of medicine, physical therapy, and lifestyle changes is frequently used to treat ankylosing spondylitis. NSAIDs, or nonsteroidal anti-inflammatory medications, are frequently used to treat pain and inflammation. Biologics have also demonstrated efficacy in the treatment of ankylosing spondylitis because they target particular pathways involved in the inflammatory process.

Ankylosing spondylitis can have a substantial impact on a person's general well-being in addition to its physical effects on the spine, such as weariness and difficulties with day-to-day functioning. Thus, for the full management of ankylosing spondylitis, a multidisciplinary strategy involving rheumatologists, physical therapists, and other medical specialists is crucial.

Managing Crystal-Induced Joint Inflammation in Gout and Other Types of Arthritis

One characteristic that sets gout apart from other forms of inflammatory arthritis is that it is linked to the buildup of urate crystals in joints, which can cause abrupt, severe pain, swelling, and redness. Although it can affect other joints as well, this ailment typically affects the joint at the base of the big toe. Apart from gout, crystal-induced inflammation is a characteristic of various other types of arthritis, such as pseudogout and hydroxyapatite crystal arthritis.

Diet, alcohol use, and obesity are among the lifestyle factors that are frequently linked to gout. Dietary changes, such as cutting out foods high in purines and drinking enough water, are essential for treating gout. Medications including urate-lowering medications and nonsteroidal anti-inflammatory drugs (NSAIDs) are frequently used to treat symptoms and stop repeated flare-ups.

In contrast, pseudogout is characterized by the accumulation of calcium pyrophosphate crystals in the joints, which produces symptoms akin to those of gout. Joint aspiration and anti-inflammatory drugs are two possible treatments for pseudogout.

Although less prevalent, hydroxyapatite crystal arthritis can result in joint discomfort and inflammation due to the deposition of hydroxyapatite crystals in joints. Medication and, in certain situations, joint suction are possible treatment options for hydroxyapatite crystal arthritis.

Comprehending the unique attributes of crystal-induced arthritis is crucial for precise diagnosis and customized treatment. Effective long-term therapy of gout and other crystal-induced forms of arthritis is ensured by regular monitoring and consultation with healthcare specialists, especially rheumatologists, even if lifestyle adjustments and drugs play a pivotal role.

CHAPTER THREE

RISK FACTORS AND CAUSES
Genetic Elements:

An individual's vulnerability to arthritis is influenced by genetic variables, which are crucial in the development of the illness. There are genetic markers and polymorphisms that have been found to raise the risk of arthritis, particularly in rheumatoid arthritis and ankylosing spondylitis cases. Due in part to these hereditary predispositions, the immune system of the body may mistakenly attack its tissues, resulting in long-term inflammation and joint damage.

For example, certain human leukocyte antigen (HLA) genes are linked to rheumatoid arthritis. Variations in these genes can raise the chance of getting rheumatoid arthritis. These genes code for proteins involved in immune system regulation. Another important component is family history; due to shared genetic features, people who have close relatives with arthritis are more likely to develop the ailment themselves.

Knowing these genetic variables helps with tailored treatment strategies as well as early detection. The intricate relationship between genetics and arthritis is still being uncovered by researchers, opening the door to more effective tailored medication that takes a patient's genetic composition into account.

Environmental Stressors:

While environmental cues act as catalysts to set off the disease in genetically predisposed individuals, genetic factors are the primary cause of arthritis. Infections, smoking, and hormone fluctuations are a few examples of environmental variables that might cause or worsen arthritic symptoms.

Certain kinds of arthritis, like reactive arthritis, have been linked to infectious agents, specifically bacteria and viruses. Inadvertently, inflammation in the joints may result from the body's immunological reaction to certain infections. In a similar vein, smoking is a major environmental risk factor for RA. Tobacco smoke contains toxic chemicals that can exacerbate immune system dysfunction and lead to the development of autoimmune diseases.

Changes in hormones are associated with the onset of arthritis, particularly in women. Hormonal changes during pregnancy or menopause, for instance, might affect how responsive the immune system is, which may lead to arthritis in people who are genetically predisposed to the condition. To stop arthritis from developing or lessen its effects, it is essential to identify and control these environmental triggers.

Joint health and arthritis:

An important role for lifestyle factors played in the onset and development of arthritis. Obesity, bad eating habits, and sedentary lifestyles increase the risk of arthritis, especially osteoarthritis. Inactivity can weaken muscles and joints, which increases the risk of developing arthritis and exacerbates symptoms already present.

Keeping up a healthy lifestyle, which includes eating a balanced diet and exercising frequently, is crucial for treating arthritis. Exercise promotes general joint health, lessens stiffness, and enhances joint function. Conversely, arthritic symptoms can be lessened by eating a diet high in anti-inflammatory foods such as fruits, vegetables, and omega-3 fatty acids.

Additionally, arthritis may develop as a result of occupational variables such as exposure to joint-stressing occupations or repeated movements. Certain occupations may make people more susceptible to joint wear and strain, which highlights the significance of workplace ergonomics and preventive measures.

Typical Risk Factors to Consider:

Several common risk factors apply to all forms of arthritis and are linked to its development. One important aspect is age: as people age, their chance of developing arthritis rises. The higher incidence of arthritis in the elderly can be attributed to a combination of factors such as aging-related joint wear and tear and the body's decreased capacity to heal injured tissues.

Gender also matters; women are more likely to get some forms of arthritis, like rheumatoid arthritis. Hormonal changes, including those associated with menopause and pregnancy, could be a factor in this gender difference. Furthermore, in general, women are more likely to develop autoimmune disorders.

One known risk factor for arthritis, especially osteoarthritis, is obesity. Being overweight puts more strain on the joints, accelerating deterioration. Preventing and treating arthritis requires maintaining a healthy weight through diet and exercise regularly.

The chance of developing arthritis in the affected joints is increased by joint trauma and injuries, which can result from sports, accidents, or repetitive stress. Injuries must be properly treated and recovered from to minimize the long-term effects on joint health.

In summary, a complete strategy to overcome arthritis must recognize and address these common risk factors in addition to an awareness of genetic and environmental impacts. Through a mix of lifestyle modifications, genetic screening, and increased knowledge, individuals can take proactive measures to prevent or manage this severe disorder.

CHAPTER FOUR

SIGNS AND CAUSES OF ILLNESS
Identifying the Signs of Arthritis

A person's quality of life can be greatly impacted by the multitude of symptoms that accompany arthritis, a complex and frequently incapacitating ailment. It is essential to identify these symptoms to provide prompt care and efficient therapy. Joint pain, which can range in intensity and be accompanied by stiffness, edema, and redness around the afflicted joints, is one of the main symptoms of arthritis. The inflammatory component of arthritis is highlighted by the fact that the pain is usually worse in the morning or after periods of inactivity.

Arthritis can have symptoms that are not limited to the joints; it can also have systemic effects. One typical symptom that may result from the body's ongoing fight against inflammation is fatigue. In addition, people with arthritis may have a decreased range of motion in their afflicted joints and muscle weakness. Because arthritis can resemble other disorders or interact with them, it can be difficult to diagnose due to its wide range of symptoms.

In addition, arthritis can strike anyone at any age, and its symptoms might appear gradually or unexpectedly. Arthritis can be a minor discomfort for some people and a life-altering affliction for others. People with arthritis and medical professionals need to be aware of the different ways the condition might present itself. A constellation of symptoms that includes joint pain, stiffness, edema, exhaustion, and limited mobility warrants consideration and research.

Certain risk factors, such as age, certain lifestyle choices, or a family history of the ailment, may occasionally be linked to arthritis. Acknowledging these risk factors in addition to the symptoms can improve the diagnosis procedure and allow for preventative strategies to control or perhaps stop the arthritis from getting worse.

The Process of Diagnosis

Because arthritis can present in a variety of ways, a thorough and multifaceted approach is necessary for making a diagnosis. Typically, medical experts start the diagnostic procedure by reviewing the patient's complete medical history to determine any potential triggers or exacerbated circumstances, as well as any trends in the symptoms and their persistence. Given that genetic predisposition can have a major impact, a family history of arthritis is particularly significant.

Physical examinations are essential for identifying range of motion, diagnosing inflammation, and evaluating joint health. Imaging tests, including magnetic resonance imaging (MRI) or X-rays, can be used to see joint structures, spot anomalies, and gauge the degree of injury. Laboratory procedures, such as joint fluid analysis and blood tests, can assist in distinguishing between various kinds of arthritis and offer important insights into the inflammatory markers.

It's crucial to remember that arthritis is a broad category of illnesses that includes, among others, psoriatic arthritis, osteoarthritis, and rheumatoid arthritis, each with specific diagnostic requirements. Therefore, developing a suitable treatment plan requires a precise diagnosis.

To guarantee an accurate diagnosis, medical professionals occasionally work with rheumatologists, experts who specialize in arthritis and related disorders.

The Value of Early Identification

Optimizing treatment outcomes and influencing the course of the disease are dependent on early identification of arthritis. Prompt action not only reduces discomfort but also lessens the likelihood of additional joint degradation. Because arthritis is inflammatory, early diagnosis is essential because untreated inflammation can result in irreparable joint damage that affects mobility and general functionality.

Early detection is important for psychological and social reasons in addition to physical health.

Living with arthritis that is misdiagnosed or untreated can lead to a lower quality of life, more stress, and anxiety. When symptoms are identified early on, people can get the help they need to get the right medical care, customized treatment programs, and lifestyle changes that can improve their general health.

Early detection also makes it easier to put disease-modifying treatments and drugs into practice, which can stop or reduce the progression of arthritis. This proactive approach treats the underlying causes of the problem in addition to mitigating its symptoms.

It also gives people with arthritis the ability to take an active role in their healthcare process, which helps them feel in control and makes them more capable of making educated decisions.

In summary, it is impossible to overestimate the importance of early detection in the context of arthritis. For those suffering from arthritis, identifying symptoms, going through a thorough diagnosis process, and starting treatments on time all work together to enhance prognosis and quality of life.

The need for early identification becomes increasingly crucial to the overall management of arthritis as medical knowledge and diagnostic capabilities continue to grow.

CHAPTER FIVE

AVAILABLE THERAPIES
Pharmaceuticals for Arthritis:

To effectively manage arthritis, a multimodal strategy is frequently used, with drugs being a key component in both symptom relief and disease progression slowing. NSAIDs, or nonsteroidal anti-inflammatory medicines, are frequently used to treat arthritis-related pain and inflammation. These drugs, which include naproxen and ibuprofen, function by preventing specific enzymes that cause inflammation. Even if they work well, long-term NSAID use carries hazards including cardiovascular problems and gastrointestinal hemorrhage.

A further family of pharmaceuticals used to treat arthritis, especially rheumatoid arthritis, are called disease-modifying antirheumatic drugs (DMARDs). One often administered DMARD that helps reduce excessive immune system activity and slow down joint degeneration is methotrexate. A more recent class of medications called biologics targets particular immune system components to further reduce inflammation. These drugs, which are frequently injected, have demonstrated encouraging outcomes in the treatment of symptoms.

Strong anti-inflammatory drugs called corticosteroids, like prednisone, may be administered for momentary alleviation during flare-ups of arthritis. However, they are usually used cautiously because of the possibility of long-term negative effects, such as immune suppression and bone loss.

For minor arthritis-related pain, acetaminophen or other painkillers may be prescribed as a substitute for NSAIDs since they reduce pain without having the same anti-inflammatory effects.

To find the best drug schedule for their particular form of arthritis, general health, and possible side effects, patients must collaborate closely with their healthcare providers.

Rehabilitation and Physical Therapy:

The comprehensive management of arthritis includes both physical therapy and rehabilitation. The goals of these therapies are to increase general mobility, lessen discomfort, and improve joint function. An expert physical therapist creates a customized exercise regimen taking into account the patient's overall health, joint involvement, and particular form of arthritis.

While strengthening exercises focus on the muscles surrounding injured joints to improve support, range of motion exercises help maintain flexibility and prevent joint stiffness. Walking or swimming are examples of aerobic workouts that can help with weight management and cardiovascular health, two things that are crucial for people with arthritis.

Physical therapists may use techniques like electrical stimulation, ultrasound, heat and cold therapy, and other modalities in addition to exercise to treat pain and inflammation. It may be suggested to use assistive equipment, like braces or splints, to support weak joints and increase functional independence.

Physical therapy aims to treat present symptoms as well as provide patients with the skills and information they need to continue exercising on their own at home. By enhancing joint health and reducing impairment, regular physical therapy sessions can considerably improve the quality of life for those with arthritis.

Surgical Procedures:

When conservative therapy is no longer effective or when joint deterioration is severe, surgery may be required for certain patients with arthritis. Joint replacement surgery, such as a hip or knee replacement, is frequently performed on individuals with arthritis who are very pained and have limited function.

Artificial metal and plastic components replace the damaged joint surfaces during joint replacement surgery. The goals of this surgical procedure are to lessen pain, restore joint function, and enhance general quality of life. Joint replacement surgeries now have higher success rates and shorter recovery times thanks to advancements in surgical techniques and implant technology.

Another surgical option for arthritis is an arthroscopy, especially if the condition is associated with inflammatory joint conditions. A tiny camera is inserted into the joint during this minimally invasive treatment to evaluate and treat a variety of joint disorders, including the removal of inflammatory synovial tissue.

Patients thinking about surgery must have a full discussion with their medical team about the advantages and disadvantages of the procedure. In most cases, post-surgical rehabilitation is necessary to maximize results and guarantee a full recovery.

Alternative & Complementary Medicines:

In addition to conventional medical treatments, complementary and alternative therapies provide other options for controlling the symptoms of arthritis. These strategies emphasize enhancing general health and mitigating pain using non-pharmacological or non-surgical means.

Tiny needles were inserted into particular body locations during the ancient Chinese art of acupuncture to enhance energy flow and reduce pain. Although acupuncture's efficacy in treating arthritis is still being studied, some patients report notable alleviation from stiffness and discomfort in their joints.

Another supplementary method that can help with these issues is massage treatment, which can also aid with circulation, flexibility, and muscle tension reduction. When administered by a qualified expert, therapeutic massage techniques may offer momentary relief from the symptoms of arthritis.

Other ways of managing arthritis are also investigated, including diet and nutritional supplements. Some people discover that making specific dietary adjustments, such as switching to an anti-inflammatory diet high in fruits, vegetables, and omega-3 fatty acids, can significantly reduce their symptoms. Furthermore, although the usefulness of supplements like glucosamine and chondroitin sulfate is still being studied, they are frequently used to maintain joint health.

Mind-body therapies, like yoga and meditation, emphasize the link between physical and mental health. For those who have arthritis, these techniques may help lower stress, promote better sleep, and improve overall quality of life.

While some people may benefit from complementary and alternative therapies, it's important to approach them with an open mind and speak with medical professionals to make sure they work well with the treatment plan as a whole. Care can be given in a more thorough and individualized way by including

these methods in a comprehensive plan for managing
arthritis.

CHAPTER SIX

LIFESTYLE MODIFICATIONS
Exercise and Arthritis:

Exercise is essential for the management of arthritis and can greatly reduce the symptoms that accompany this illness. Despite popular belief, physical activity is not harmful to people with arthritis; on the contrary, it is an essential part of a successful arthritis management strategy. Frequent exercise enhances flexibility, strengthens the muscles around afflicted joints, and preserves joint function. Walking, cycling, and swimming are examples of low-impact exercises that are frequently advised because they reduce joint stress and improve cardiovascular health.

Additionally, physiotherapists or medical specialists can create customized workout regimens that target particular joint locations to accommodate the demands and limitations of each individual. To improve total joint health, these programs usually combine strength training, stretching, and aerobic exercises. Crucially, to prevent overexertion, people with arthritis should aim for a balanced and moderate approach. Consistency is essential.

Exercise has many physical advantages, but it also helps with weight management, which is important for managing arthritis. Sustaining a healthy weight eases pain and delays the advancement of arthritis by lessening the strain on weight-bearing joints like the knees and hips.

Arthritis and Nutrition:

When it comes to managing arthritis, nutrition is essential because it affects both preventing the condition and reducing its symptoms. Joint health and general well-being can be enhanced by eating a varied, well-balanced diet. Omega-3 fatty acids, which are present in walnuts, flaxseeds, and fish oil, have anti-inflammatory qualities and may help arthritis sufferers experience less stiffness and discomfort in their joints.

Fruits and vegetables, which are high in antioxidants, can also be very helpful in treating arthritis by scavenging free radicals that cause inflammation. Furthermore, bone health must maintain an adequate amount of vitamin D, and attaining optimal levels can be facilitated by exposure to sunlight and dietary sources such as fortified meals and fatty fish.

It is crucial to remember that everyone's reaction to a given dish may differ. Certain diets, such as those heavy in processed sugars and saturated fats, can cause inflammation. Some people with arthritis may find relief by eliminating these foods. A diet plan that suits a person's needs and tastes can be customized with the assistance of a nutritionist or other healthcare professional.

Techniques for Stress Management:

Effective stress management strategies are essential for people with arthritis because stress is believed to worsen the symptoms of the condition. Stress can exacerbate pain and inflammation, making arthritis more difficult to manage daily. Deep breathing exercises, yoga, and meditation are examples of relaxation practices that can be used to lessen the negative effects of stress on the body and mind.

Cognitive-behavioral therapy (CBT) is an additional useful tool for arthritic stress management. Through the identification and modification of negative thought patterns, this treatment method helps people cultivate a more positive outlook and lower their stress levels. A general sense of well-being can also be enhanced by partaking in enjoyable and calming activities, such as hobbies, time spent in nature, or interacting with loved ones.

Furthermore, implementing time management techniques and establishing attainable objectives helps lessen the psychological strain sometimes connected to long-term ailments like arthritis. Through multifaceted stress management, people can enhance their quality of life and effectively manage the difficulties associated with arthritis.

The Function of Sleep in the Management of Arthritis:

Good sleep is important for everyone, but it's especially important for people with arthritis. The body's healing processes depend heavily on sleep, and inadequate or disturbed sleep can aggravate the pain and exhaustion associated with arthritis. Developing healthy sleeping habits can make a big difference in how arthritis is managed overall.

Good sleep hygiene includes practicing relaxation techniques before bedtime, keeping a regular sleep schedule, and furnishing a cozy sleeping space. People with arthritis must find a comfortable sleeping posture that reduces joint tension. A mattress with sufficient support and the use of supportive pillows or cushions can significantly improve the quality of your sleep.

It's also very important to take care of pain management before going to bed. This could include using heat or cold therapy to relieve sore joints or following a doctor's instructions on taking prescribed drugs. The body can be signaled to slow down by a relaxing nighttime routine, including reading or light stretching, which can make the transition into restful sleep easier.

Creating a holistic strategy for managing arthritis requires an understanding of how nutrition, exercise, stress reduction, and sleep are all related. People can better manage the difficulties brought on by arthritis and enhance their general well-being by adopting these lifestyle changes into their everyday lives.

CHAPTER SEVEN

WORKING TOGETHER WITH MEDICAL EXPERTS
Putting Together a Helpful Medical Team

Building a supportive healthcare team is essential to the fight against arthritis. Because arthritis is a complex disorder, several healthcare experts must work together to address its varied elements. Physical therapists, occupational therapists, rheumatologists, and orthopedic specialists usually make up this core group. Everybody adds a different set of skills to the overall strategy for controlling arthritis.

When it comes to arthritis diagnosis and treatment, rheumatologists are crucial. These specialist doctors are equipped with the knowledge to determine the precise kind of arthritis a patient may have and create a customized course of care. Working together with orthopedic doctors, they guarantee a comprehensive approach that includes surgery when needed. Efficient communication between healthcare providers is crucial for precise diagnosis, prompt treatment, and continuous supervision.

Physical therapists must be included in addition to medical professionals to promote a comprehensive approach to arthritis management. Enhancing mobility, strength, and flexibility is the specialty of physical therapists, who customize exercise regimens to meet each patient's specific demands and limits. Rheumatologists, orthopedic specialists, and physical therapists work together to address the limits imposed by arthritis as well as the underlying medical issues in a synergistic manner.

Occupational therapists are another member of the support team who helps people adjust to daily tasks despite the difficulties caused by arthritis. Occupational therapists collaborate closely with patients to create workable plans for dressing, cooking, and other daily duties. People with arthritis can keep their independence in their everyday activities and improve their quality of life by incorporating the knowledge of occupational therapists into their healthcare team.

Creating a healthcare team that is supportive to overcome arthritis is a team effort that utilizes the special abilities of different professionals. The collaborative efforts of rheumatologists, orthopedic experts, physical therapists, and occupational therapists guarantee a thorough and individualized management strategy for arthritis, encompassing the functional and medical dimensions of the ailment.

Efficient Interaction with Physicians and Experts

The key to managing arthritis successfully is effective communication. To guarantee that patients receive the best care possible and that medical personnel are aware of the patient's experiences and concerns, it is crucial to establish open and transparent channels of communication with doctors and specialists.

Patients should, above all, feel empowered to discuss their symptoms, difficulties, and objectives with their doctors during consultations.

Clear communication about the type and degree of pain, functional restrictions, and impact on day-to-day functioning gives medical professionals important information for precise diagnosis and treatment planning. Patients' diaries can be a useful tool for recording changes and trends, which can lead to better-informed discussions during visits.

On the other hand, medical personnel should use active listening techniques to understand the subtleties of the patient's arthritic experience. Establishing a compassionate and nonjudgmental atmosphere cultivates trust, allowing patients to freely express their worries. Additionally, to encourage patients and healthcare professionals to participate in joint decision-making, physicians and specialists should clearly and understandably convey treatment alternatives, possible side effects, and the long-term prognosis.

Additionally, technology can be a key factor in improving communication. Platforms for telemedicine make it possible for patients and medical experts to consult remotely, facilitating continuous communication—particularly during periods when in-person visits may be difficult. Virtual or in-person, routine follow-ups allow physicians to track the effectiveness of their treatment, make any necessary modifications, and quickly address any new problems.

Essentially, the key to beating arthritis is good communication between patients and medical staff. By ensuring that patients receive individualized care and keeping physicians and specialists informed about the condition's shifting nature, this two-way communication eventually supports a cooperative and effective management strategy.

Occupational and Physical Therapists' Role

Occupational and physical therapists are essential to the overall care of patients with arthritis. Their knowledge goes beyond treating patients medically;

instead, they concentrate on improving their mobility, functionality, and general quality of life.

Physical therapists play a crucial role in creating exercise plans that are customized to the unique requirements and limits of individuals with arthritis. These exercises are designed to strengthen muscles, reduce discomfort, and increase joint flexibility. Physical therapists work closely with rheumatologists and orthopedic experts to make sure that exercise regimens are in line with the aims of medical treatment and do not worsen underlying conditions. Patients benefit physically from regular visits with a physical therapist, but they also provide an opportunity for continual evaluation and modification of the treatment plan.

Conversely, occupational therapists concentrate on the functional components of daily living that are impacted by arthritis. To support independent living, they advise patients on assistive technology and collaborate with them to create adaptive solutions. Occupational therapists play a major role in the functional aspects of arthritis therapy, offering advice on everything from workplace ergonomic changes to energy-saving measures for everyday tasks.

Combined efforts by occupational and physical therapists are especially noticeable in full-service rehabilitation programs. These programs are designed to meet the multifaceted issues that arthritis poses and are frequently created in cooperation with orthopedic and rheumatology specialists. Patients can reclaim control over their lives by utilizing a combination of joint protection techniques, adaptive strategies, and rehabilitative exercises.

To sum up, the functions of occupational and physical therapists are essential to the comprehensive treatment of arthritis. Their joint efforts with other medical specialists result in a comprehensive strategy that takes into account the functional as well as the medical aspects of the illness, enabling patients to live happy, fulfilled lives despite the difficulties caused by arthritis.

CHAPTER EIGHT

ADAPTIVE TECHNIQUES
Arthritis's Effect on Emotions:

Chronic arthritis, which is defined as inflammation of the joints, hurts people's mental and physical health in addition to their physical health. Arthritis can have a significant emotional impact, resulting in emotions such as irritation, worry, and depression. Living with arthritis's ongoing pain and restrictions can make people feel as though they've lost something since they can't do the things they used to enjoy. Emotional anguish is made worse by the unpredictable nature of flare-ups, which results in an ongoing sense of uncertainty.

Getting used to a new reality is one of the biggest emotional challenges. Patients frequently struggle with the emotional roller coaster that comes with embracing a chronic illness that may have different effects on their everyday lives.

Overwhelming feelings of powerlessness and lack of control are possible. Furthermore, it's important to recognize the significant influence arthritis has on self-esteem because physical manifestations of the disease, including joint abnormalities, can cause issues with body image and social isolation.

Handling the psychological effects of arthritis calls for a comprehensive strategy. Through psychoeducation, counseling, and the creation of coping mechanisms, emotional well-being can be fostered. Addressing the emotional aspects of arthritis requires open communication with healthcare providers and the creation of a supportive atmosphere at home. Involving friends and family in the process can also assist people in negotiating the difficulties and emotional upheavals that frequently accompany this chronic condition by offering emotional support.

Patient and caregiver coping strategies:

Arthritis requires a multimodal strategy that includes practical, psychological, and physical coping mechanisms. Taking the initiative to manage the disease is a crucial coping tool. This entails remaining up to date on arthritis, comprehending available treatments, and actively engaging in healthcare decision-making. Acquiring knowledge empowers patients by improving their coping skills and giving them a sense of control over their health.

Lifestyle changes are a common component of physical coping techniques. Exercise that is customized for each person's needs and tastes can help keep muscles and joints strong and flexible. Incorporating stress-reduction methods like yoga or meditation, controlling weight, and keeping a balanced diet all contribute to general well-being. In addition to helping with everyday chores, adaptive tools and assistive technologies can lessen the physical strain that comes with having arthritis.

Resilience building and having an optimistic outlook are essential emotional coping mechanisms. Emotional coping is built on acceptance of the condition and concentrating on what can be accomplished rather than dwelling on limits. Despite the difficulties caused by arthritis, mental health can be greatly enhanced by partaking in joyful and fulfilling activities.

Caregivers have an equally challenging job in supporting patients with arthritis. It is essential to cultivate understanding, empathy, and patience. To avoid burnout, caregivers can profit by looking for their support systems, using educational resources, and making sure they prioritize self-care. Open communication creates a shared knowledge of the difficulties and encourages a team approach to managing arthritis. This is especially true for patients and caregivers.

Resources and Support Groups:

Understanding the value of having a strong support network, several tools and support groups have been developed to help those living with arthritis. These support groups are essential for exchanging stories, offering emotional support, and giving useful guidance on how to manage the illness.

Individuals facing comparable issues come together in local and virtual support groups, fostering a feeling of camaraderie and comprehension. Through these forums, users can share coping mechanisms, talk about available treatments, and learn how to get past the obstacles that arthritis presents daily. Furthermore, support groups provide a forum for people to freely express their feelings, which lessens the feeling of loneliness that frequently accompanies long-term illnesses.

In addition to peer support, there are a plethora of tools available to educate and empower people with arthritis. Reputable arthritis foundations organize workshops, online resources, and educational materials that offer important knowledge about arthritis, treatment alternatives, and lifestyle management. Having access to these resources improves understanding and gives people the means to take an active role in their healthcare journey.

To sum up, resources and support groups serve as pillars of strength for people with arthritis, encouraging a sense of empowerment, shared understanding, and community. These paths make a substantial contribution to the all-encompassing strategy required to successfully manage the difficulties presented by arthritis.

CHAPTER NINE

INVESTIGATIONS AND NOVELTIES
Present Advances in the Study of Arthritis:

Millions of people worldwide are impacted by arthritis, a chronic illness that is defined by joint inflammation. Current directions in arthritis research have moved toward a comprehensive picture of the condition that takes into account lifestyle, genetic, environmental, and physiological elements of the illness.

Uncovering the intricate genetic causes of arthritis is a popular area of study, and advances in genomics have made it possible for scientists to pinpoint particular gene mutations linked to a higher risk of developing the condition. This information paves the way for customized medicine, which will enable individualized treatment plans based on a patient's genetic makeup.

Moreover, the involvement of the microbiome in the development of arthritis is gaining more and more attention from researchers. Studies are being conducted to find out how changes in the composition of the gut microbiome may influence the pathophysiology of arthritis. In particular, the gut microbiota has been connected to immune system modulation. This new method not only broadens our knowledge of the condition but also opens the door for creative therapeutic approaches that target the gut microbiota to reduce arthritic symptoms.

Apart from these studies that focus on genes and microbiomes, there is an increasing emphasis on examining the role of lifestyle variables in arthritis. It is now known that a person's diet, level of activity, and stress management are important factors that can either make their arthritis symptoms worse or better. Extensive research is being conducted to clarify the precise food habits and exercise routines that might support joint health, offering patients evidence-based lifestyle suggestions as part of an all-encompassing arthritis treatment strategy.

Innovative technologies for monitoring arthritis have also been developed through collaboration between researchers and IT developers. Sensor-equipped wearables can track joint mobility, giving medical professionals and patients useful information. These technology developments facilitate early flare-up identification and optimize treatment regimens, allowing for a more proactive and individualized approach to managing arthritis.

New Medical Procedures and Technology:

The advent of novel medicines and technologies is bringing about a radical change in the management of arthritis. One significant advancement is the creation of biologic medications, which specifically target immune system components that cause inflammation in cases of arthritis. Patients with rheumatoid arthritis and other autoimmune forms of the disease now have new hope thanks to the amazing efficacy of these medications, such as TNF-alpha inhibitors, in lowering joint inflammation and delaying the course of the ailment.

Furthermore, regenerative medicine has the potential to completely transform the way that arthritis is treated. Injections of platelet-rich plasma and stem cell therapies are intended to encourage tissue regeneration and repair, providing a potential remedy for the damaged cartilage linked to arthritis. Positive outcomes from early clinical trials suggest that regenerative medicine may be a major factor in the treatment of arthritis in the future.

Treatment options for arthritis are also being influenced by developments in precision medicine. More focused and efficient treatments are possible when treatment plans are customized according to each patient's distinct genetic composition and illness profile. This individualized method represents a major advancement toward more effective and patient-centered care by improving treatment outcomes and minimizing side effects.

Artificial intelligence (AI) is revolutionizing the field of technology by greatly advancing the diagnosis and treatment of arthritis. AI systems can recognize trends and forecast the course of disease by analyzing large, complicated datasets, such as patient records and medical imaging. This promotes a more proactive and individualized approach to arthritis care by enabling early intervention and the optimization of treatment strategies.

In conclusion, a multimodal strategy that incorporates genetic discoveries, lifestyle factors, and technological advancements is reflected in the changing landscape of arthritis research and therapy. In the continuous fight against this crippling illness, these developments not only broaden our understanding of arthritis but also open up new possibilities for patient-friendly, tailored, and more successful interventions.

CHAPTER TEN

PREVENTIVE AND UPKEEP
Lifestyle Modifications to Prevent Arthritis:

It is crucial to live a proactive, health-conscious lifestyle when it comes to preventing arthritis. A key component of this lifestyle is regular exercise, which has a major positive impact on joint health. Walking, cycling, and swimming are examples of low-impact exercises that can help preserve joint flexibility and lower the risk of arthritis.

Furthermore, it's imperative to keep a healthy weight because extra weight puts undue strain on joints, especially the knees and hips, which carry a lot of weight. An equally important diet is both well-balanced and nutrient-rich since some foods have anti-inflammatory qualities that help relieve joint pain and lower the chance of developing arthritis.

One crucial but frequently overlooked aspect of preventing arthritis is stress management. Prolonged stress can worsen inflammation and be a factor in joint pain, so it's critical to include stress-relieving activities like yoga, meditation, or deep breathing exercises in daily life. It is also imperative that you get enough sleep to maintain a healthy lifestyle. In addition to impairing immunity, inadequate sleep can exacerbate inflammation, which may lead to arthritis or exacerbate pre-existing conditions.

Additional lifestyle decisions that can have a big impact on preventing arthritis include abstaining from tobacco and consuming alcohol in moderation. Smoking has been connected to a higher risk of developing rheumatoid arthritis, and drinking too much alcohol can impair the body's capacity to absorb vital nutrients, which can harm joints. People can strengthen their defenses against arthritis and create an atmosphere that supports general joint health by adopting certain lifestyle changes.

Frequent Health Examinations and Monitoring:

Regular medical examinations are essential for the early diagnosis and treatment of arthritis. The monitoring of important indicators, such as joint function, inflammatory levels, and general musculoskeletal health, is made possible by routine visits to healthcare providers. These examinations allow for prompt intervention and the application of preventive measures, which may stop the advancement of arthritis or lessen its effects.

Diagnostic procedures, such as blood tests and imaging investigations, are essential parts of physical examinations for the monitoring of arthritis. Blood testing can identify particular markers linked to different forms of arthritis, offering important information on the underlying pathophysiology of joint pain. Imaging methods, such as magnetic resonance imaging (MRI) and X-rays, aid in the visualization of joint structures and the detection of any abnormalities or injuries.

People who are at risk of arthritis or who have a family history of the disease should be proactive in keeping an eye on their health in addition to routine check-ups. Being aware of even the most minute alterations in joint function, including pain, swelling, or stiffness, enables early intervention and can stop arthritis from worsening. Regularly evaluating oneself and keeping lines of communication open with medical professionals foster a team-based approach to managing arthritis, guaranteeing that new problems are identified and resolved quickly.

Strategies for Long-Term Maintenance:

The foundation of long-term maintenance treatments for arthritis is a thorough and multidimensional approach to controlling the disease throughout time. The foundation of these tactics is physical therapy, which emphasizes activities that increase mobility overall, strengthen surrounding muscles, and improve joint flexibility. When it comes to treating any functional limitations and customizing exercises to meet the unique needs of each individual, the advice of a qualified physical therapist is important.

To maintain arthritis in the long term, medication management is frequently essential. Pain management, inflammation reduction, and disease progression slowing are common goals of prescribing biologics, DMARDs, and nonsteroidal anti-inflammatory medications (NSAIDs). Frequent medication reviews with medical professionals guarantee that the treatment plan is still effective and can be modified as necessary.

Long-term arthritis management still heavily relies on leading a healthy lifestyle in addition to taking drugs and receiving physical therapy. Maintaining a healthy, well-balanced diet rich in anti-inflammatory foods, engaging in physical activity only to the extent comfortable for each individual, and controlling stress are all lifelong practices that enhance well-being. Scheduling routine follow-up consultations with healthcare experts to evaluate the progression of the disease and make necessary adjustments to treatment regimens guarantees that management techniques stay in line with the changing demands of people with arthritis. Essentially, the secret to long-term maintenance is a customized, all-encompassing strategy that prioritizes the patient's quality of life while addressing the dynamic character of arthritis.

CHAPTER ELEVEN

ACHIEVEMENTS
Actual Accounts of People Overcoming Arthritis:

Arthritis can have a severe influence on a person's quality of life, and its devastating effects affect countless people worldwide. Nevertheless, despite the difficulties associated with arthritis, there are encouraging accounts of people who have overcome the condition under the supervision of medical professionals. These first-hand accounts offer hope to individuals who are now struggling with the negative effects of arthritis.

One such tale is that of Sarah, who developed rheumatoid arthritis at the age of 45 and was left crippled by pain and stiffness. Exasperated with the restrictions the illness placed on her day-to-day activities, Sarah consulted a rheumatologist, who customized an extensive course of treatment. Sarah increasingly recovered control over her life by combining physical treatment, medicine, and lifestyle changes. Her experience serves as a powerful example of the critical role that professional advice plays in recognizing the individuality of each patient's situation and customizing treatment options.

Michael's story, a retired athlete with osteoarthritis, is another powerful one. Fearing that his active lifestyle would be gone forever, Michael sought advice from a group of medical professionals, including physical therapists and orthopedic surgeons. He successfully had a joint replacement surgery and started a rehabilitation program that not only improved his mobility but also revived his love of exercise under their direction. Michael's tale demonstrates the life-changing power of professional guidance in discovering cutting-edge therapies and restoring a sense of normalcy.

The significance of early intervention and cooperative efforts between patients and healthcare professionals is a recurring topic in these memoirs. All varieties of arthritis necessitate a multimodal strategy that extends beyond medication; this approach frequently includes dietary modifications, exercise routines, and psychological support. Acquiring a meaningful life following arthritis necessitates dedication to obtaining professional advice and actively engaging in the therapeutic process.

Inspirational Travels with Skilled Advice:

Overcoming arthritis is a deep and life-changing event rather than just a medical procedure. The experiences of those who have successfully traveled this journey under the direction of experts serve as monuments to the human spirit's tenacity and the value of patients and healthcare providers working together.

James's story is one of perseverance in the face of psoriatic arthritis. Under the supervision of a rheumatologist who specializes in autoimmune diseases, James investigated a holistic treatment plan. Through therapy and support groups, his expert-guided path addressed the emotional toll of chronic illness in addition to managing the physical symptoms. James recovered to be both mentally and physically stronger, demonstrating the critical role that professional supervision plays in addressing the overall health and well-being of arthritis patients.

Maria's experience with juvenile idiopathic arthritis serves as an example of how crucial pediatric rheumatologists are in offering specialized therapy. Together with her medical team, Maria's parents worked closely to create a treatment plan that was specifically customized for her. With the help of physical therapy, educational assistance, and medication modifications, Maria was able to control her symptoms and achieve academic success. Her moving story highlights the significant influence of professional advice in determining the course of adolescent arthritis patients' lives.

These travel experiences highlight the value of an individualized and all-encompassing strategy for managing arthritis. Expert coaching goes beyond clinical factors to include knowledge of the patient's goals, lifestyle, and mental health. With the assistance of skilled medical professionals, people must work together to overcome the challenges presented by arthritis in a resilient and determined manner. The ensuing success stories provide hope to people who are currently dealing with the difficulties posed by arthritis by showing that an active and full life is not only feasible but attainable with the correct support.

THE END

www.ingramcontent.com/pod-product-compliance
Lightning Source LLC
Chambersburg PA
CBHW050743260726

48661CB00001B/391